Taking Care of Myself

Eating Right

By Meg Gaertner

level 2 little blue readers

www.littlebluehousebooks.com

Little Blue House is distributed by North Star Editions:
sales@northstareditions.com | 888-417-0195

Produced for Little Blue House by Red Line Editorial.

Photographs ©: Shutterstock Images, cover, 4, 6–7, 9, 10 (top), 10 (bottom), 13 (top), 13 (bottom), 14–15, 21 (top), 22, 24 (top left), 24 (top right), 24 (bottom left), 24 (bottom right); iStockphoto, 17, 18–19, 21 (bottom)

Library of Congress Control Number: 2021916808

ISBN
978-1-64619-490-2 (hardcover)
978-1-64619-517-6 (paperback)
978-1-64619-568-8 (ebook pdf)
978-1-64619-544-2 (hosted ebook)

Printed in the United States of America
Mankato, MN
012022

About the Author

Meg Gaertner enjoys reading, writing, dancing, and being outside. She lives in Minnesota.

Table of Contents

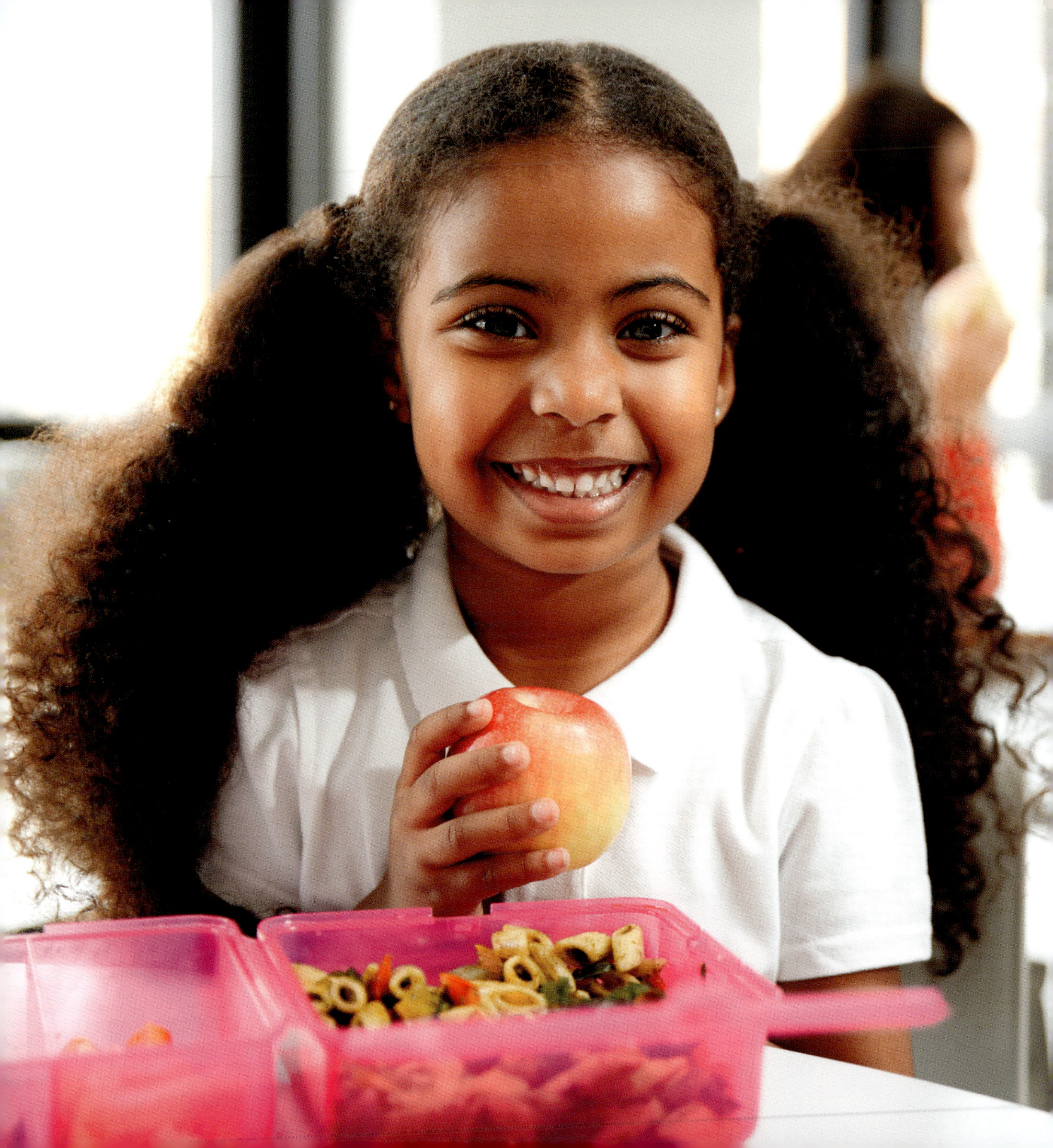

Energy and Nutrients

Food gives people energy. Different foods have different nutrients. Nutrients are things that keep the body healthy.

Some nutrients help people see.

Some help the body heal.

Some help the body get stronger.

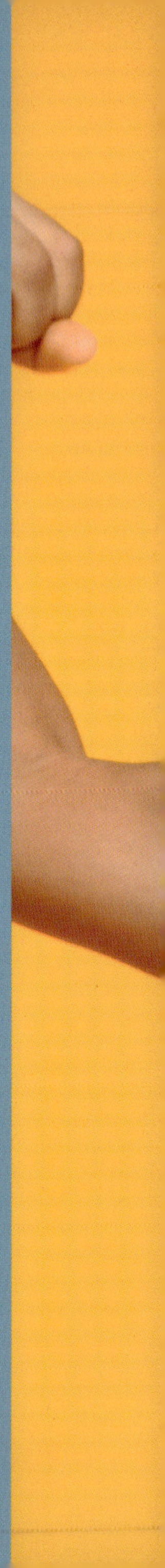

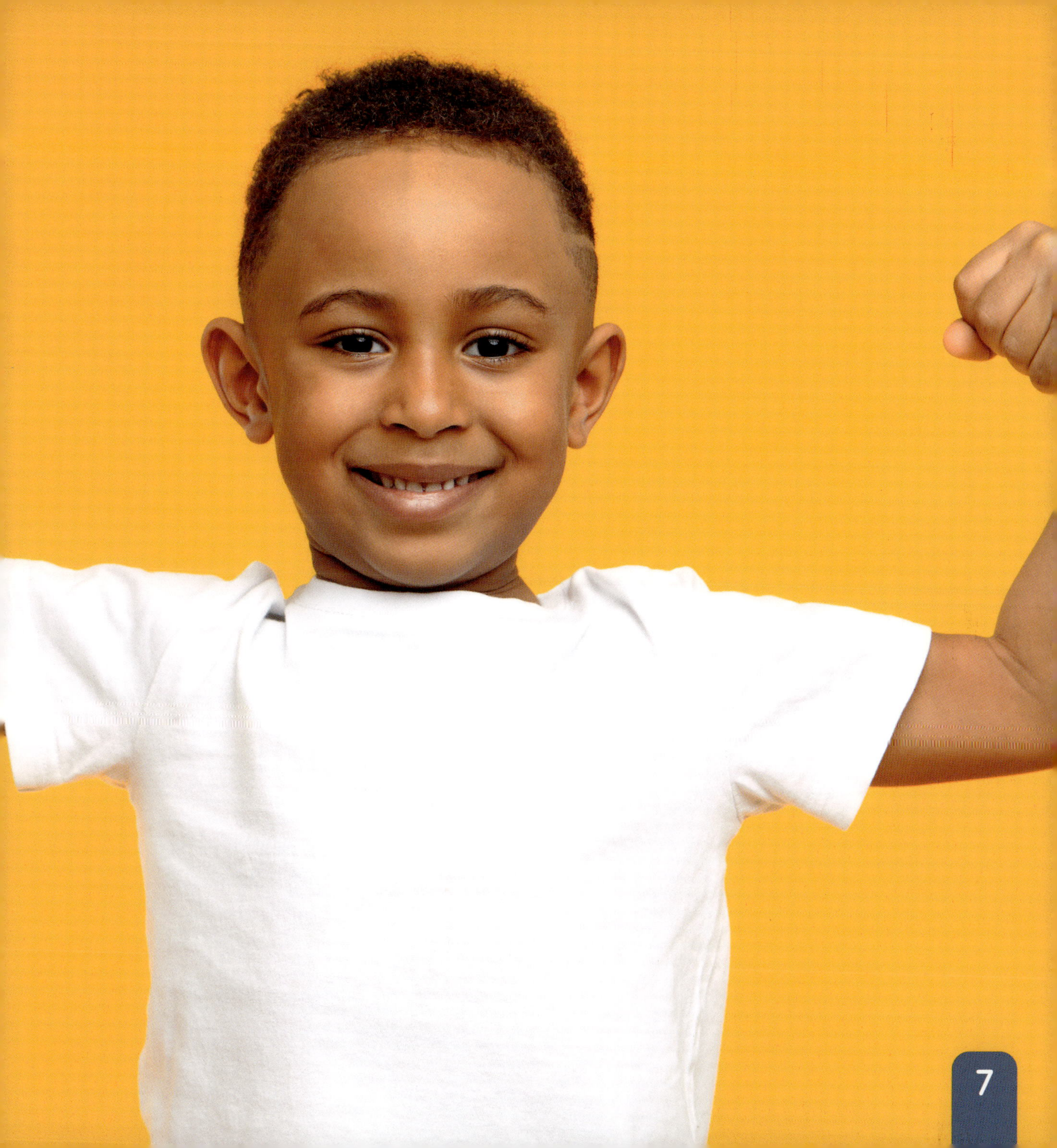

It's good to eat many different kinds of food. That way, you get all the nutrients your body needs.

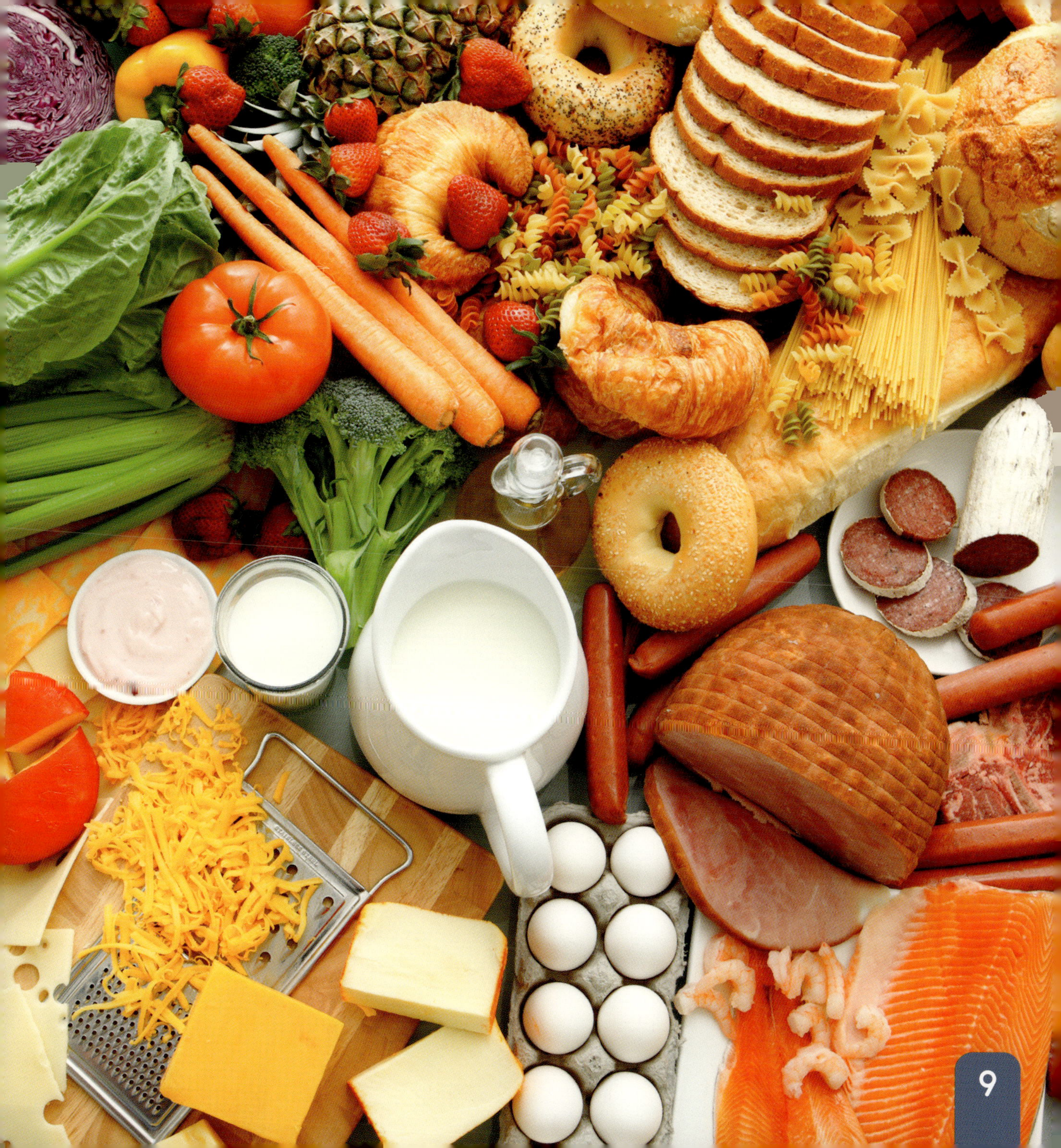

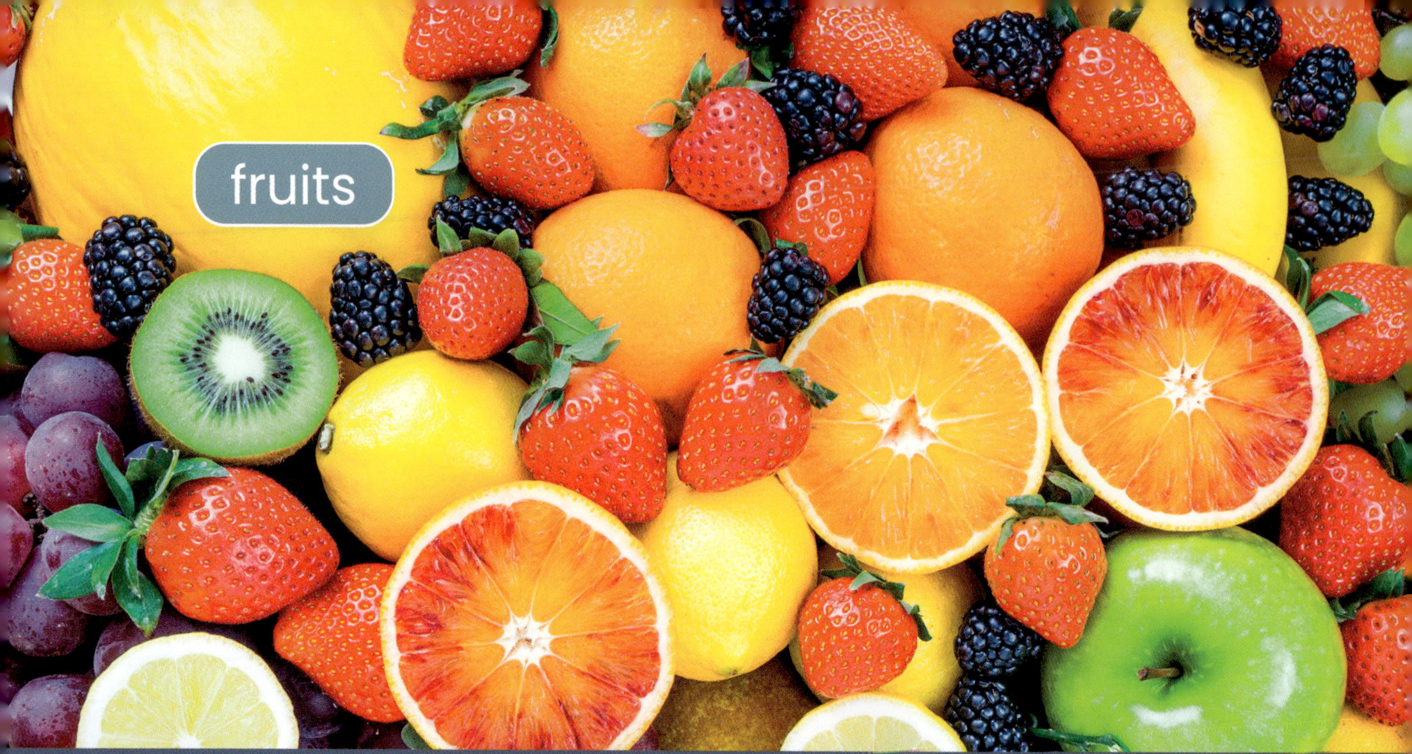
fruits

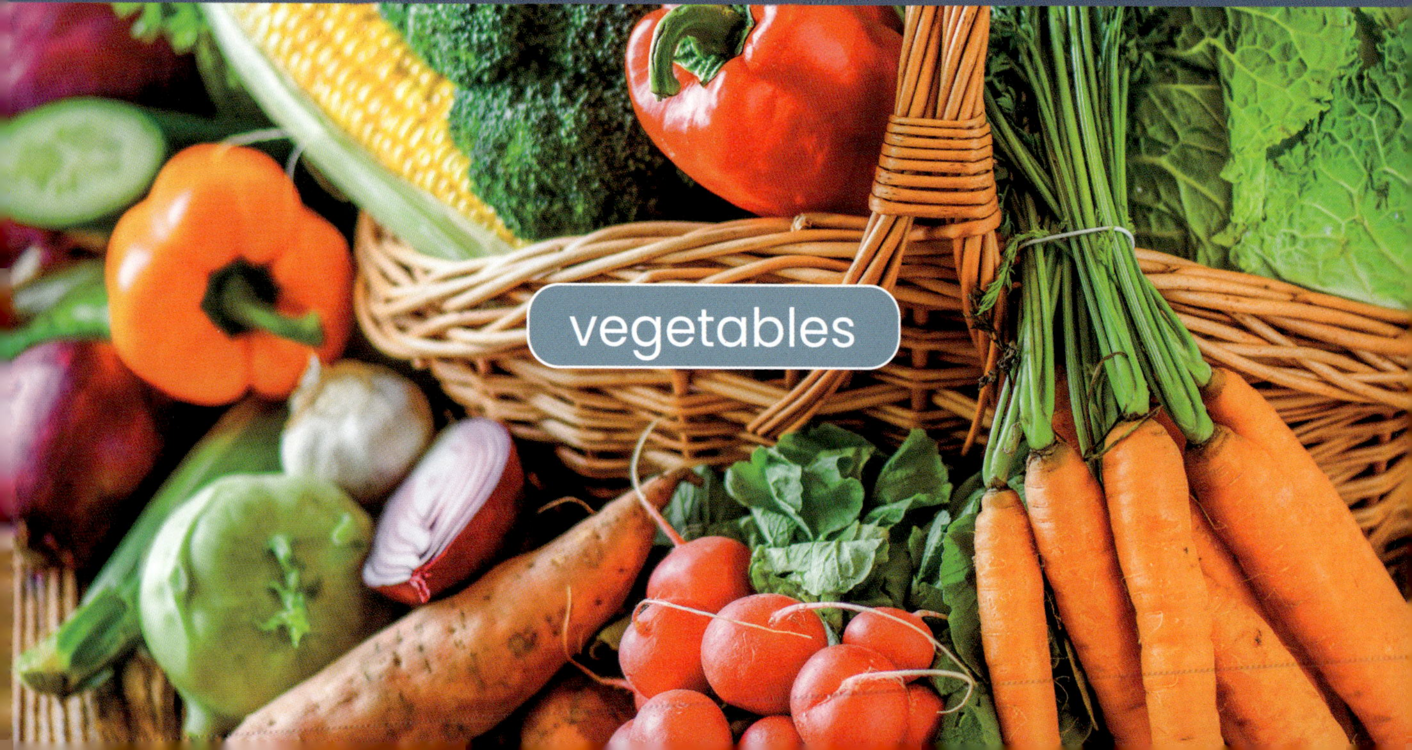
vegetables

Kinds of Food

Fruits and vegetables are healthy foods.
They have many nutrients.
People should eat them with every meal.

For example, add berries to your cereal at breakfast. Pack carrots in your lunch box. Have an apple for a snack. Eat cooked green beans at dinner.

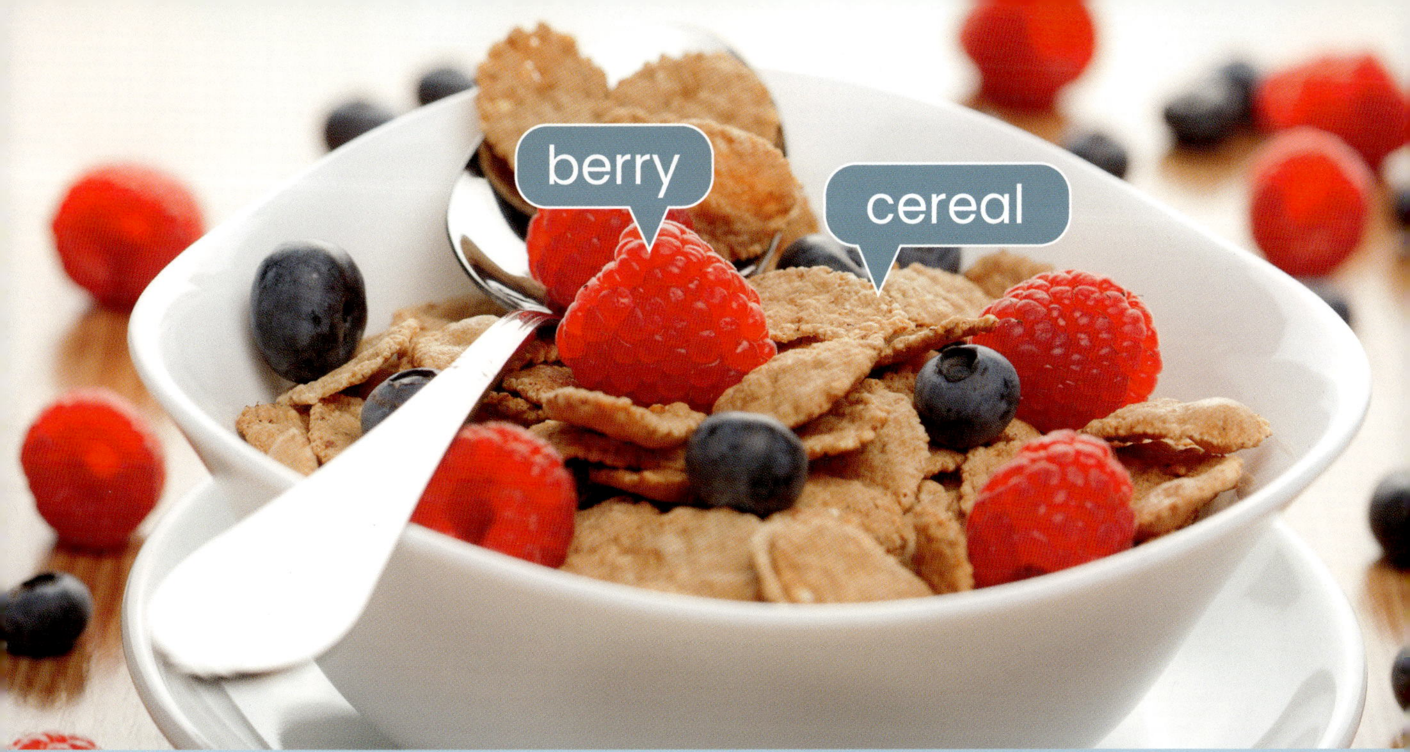
berry
cereal

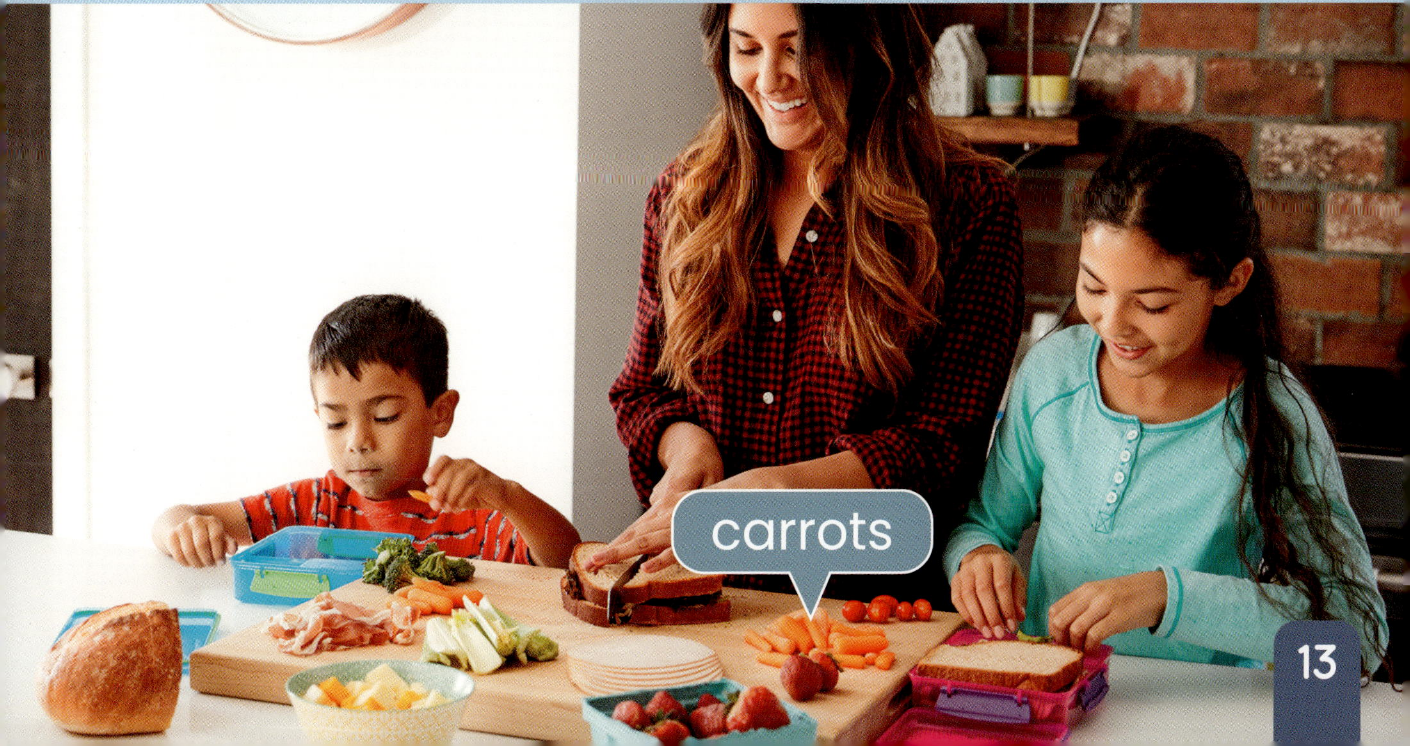
carrots

Grains have many nutrients, too. Grains include bread, rice, and pasta. They help people feel full. That way, people are less likely to eat too much.

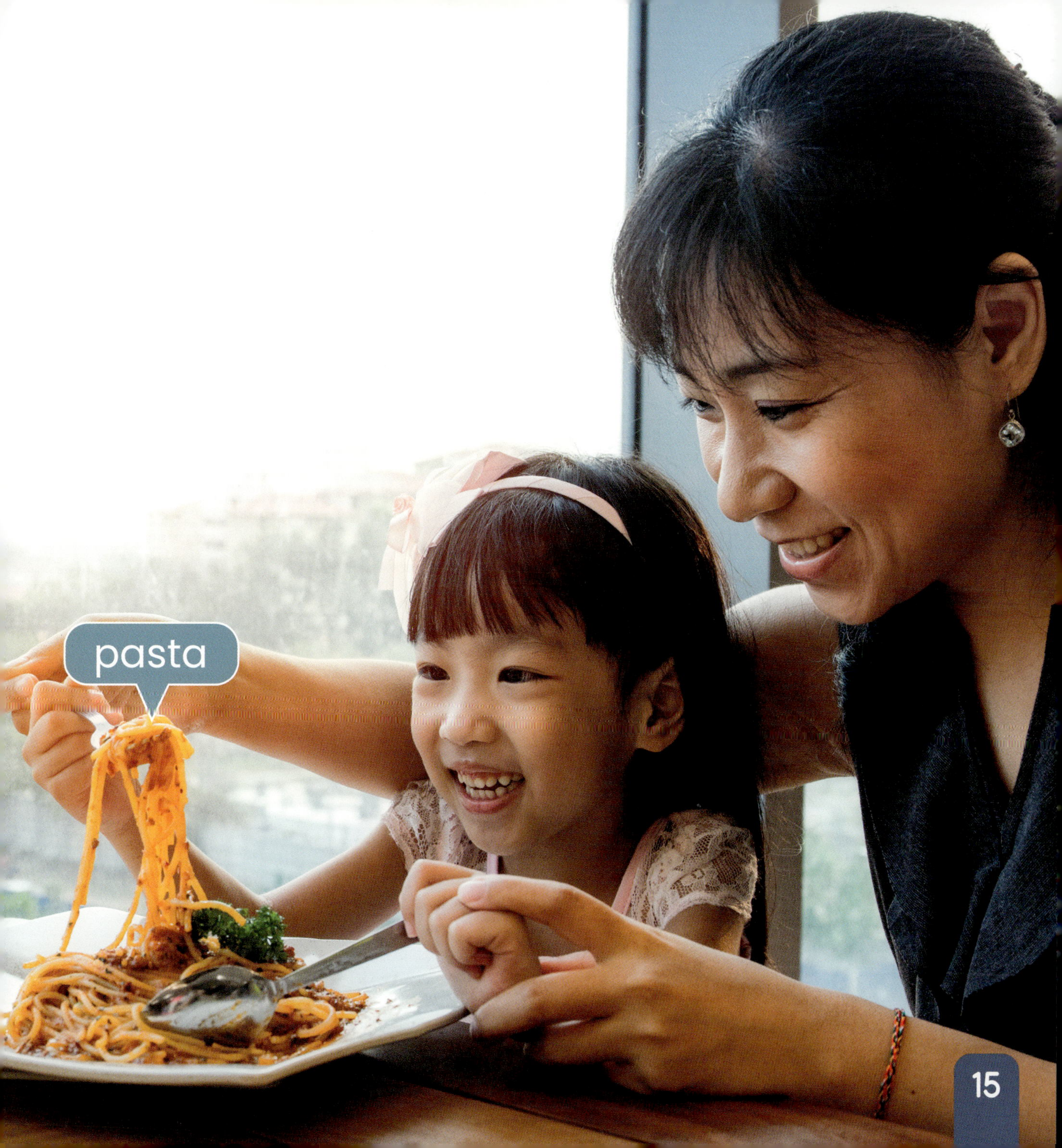
pasta

Protein is great for energy.
It also helps strengthen
the body.
Fish and eggs
have protein.
Beans and nuts do, too.

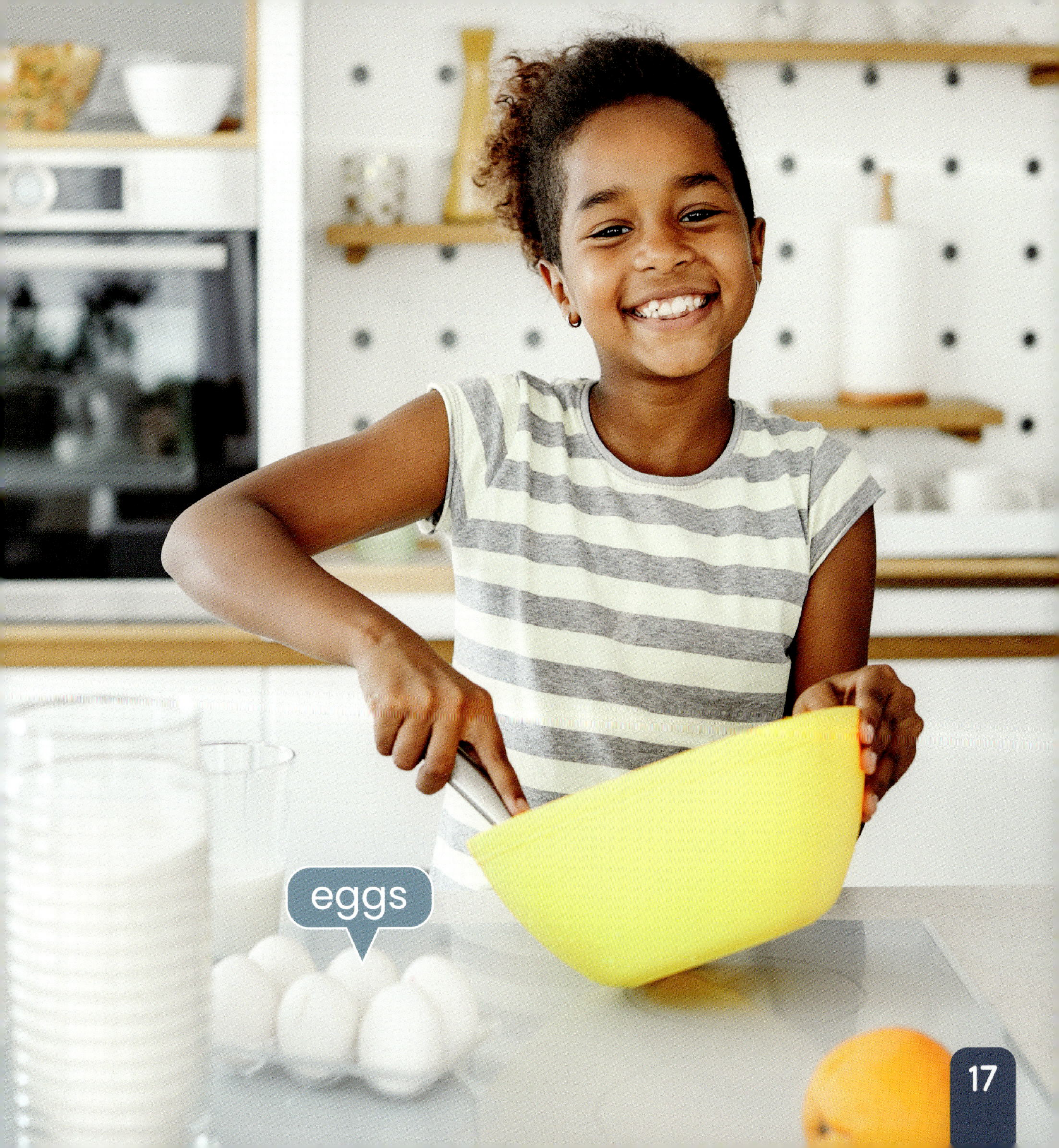
eggs

Some foods are healthier than others. For example, it's okay to eat ice cream sometimes. But don't eat it every day. It doesn't have many nutrients.

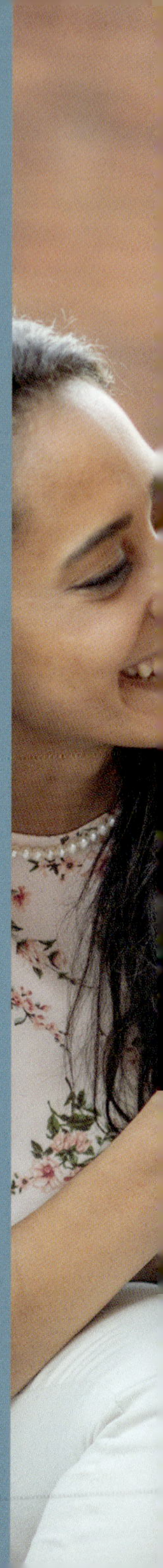

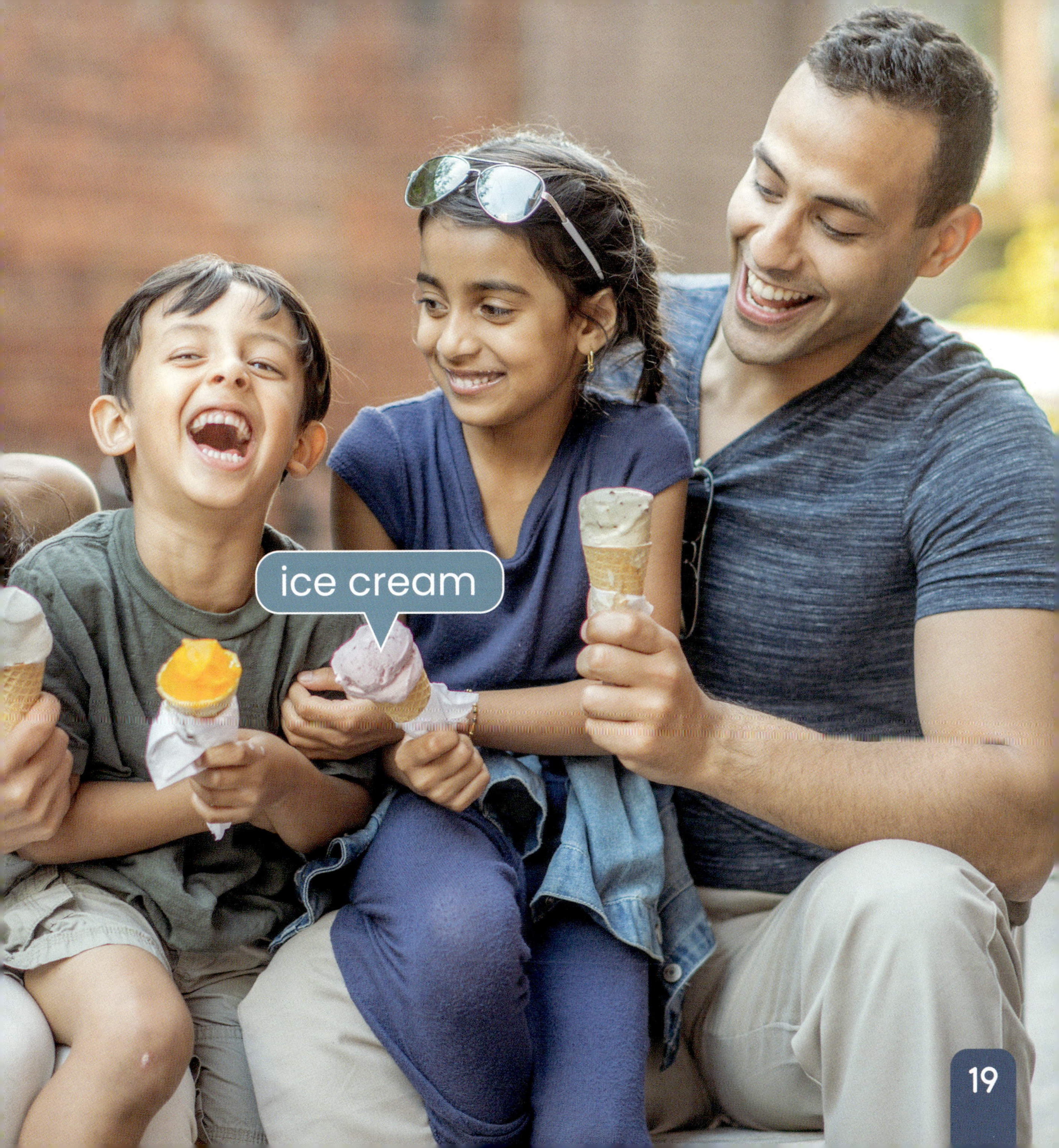
ice cream

Drinking right is important, too. The body needs water to survive, so drink lots of water. Avoid sodas and other sugary drinks.

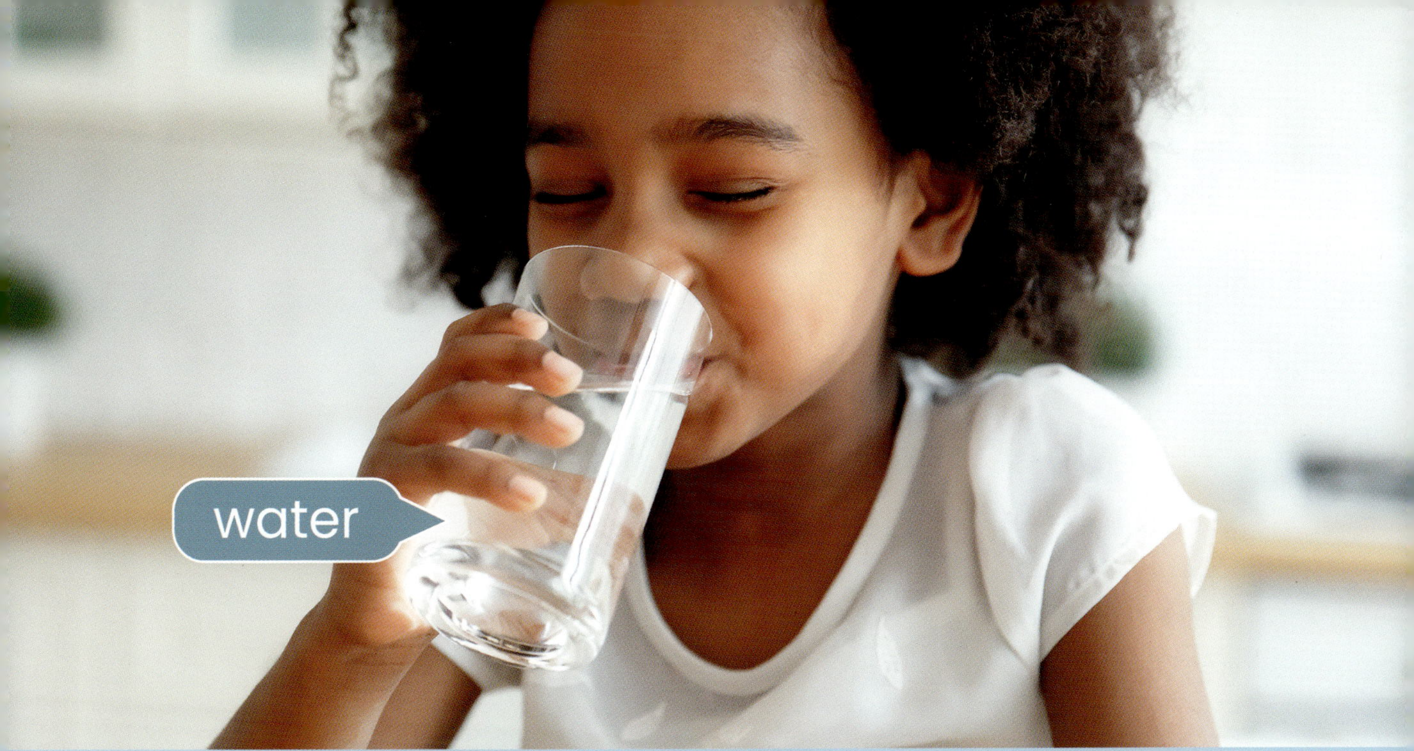
water

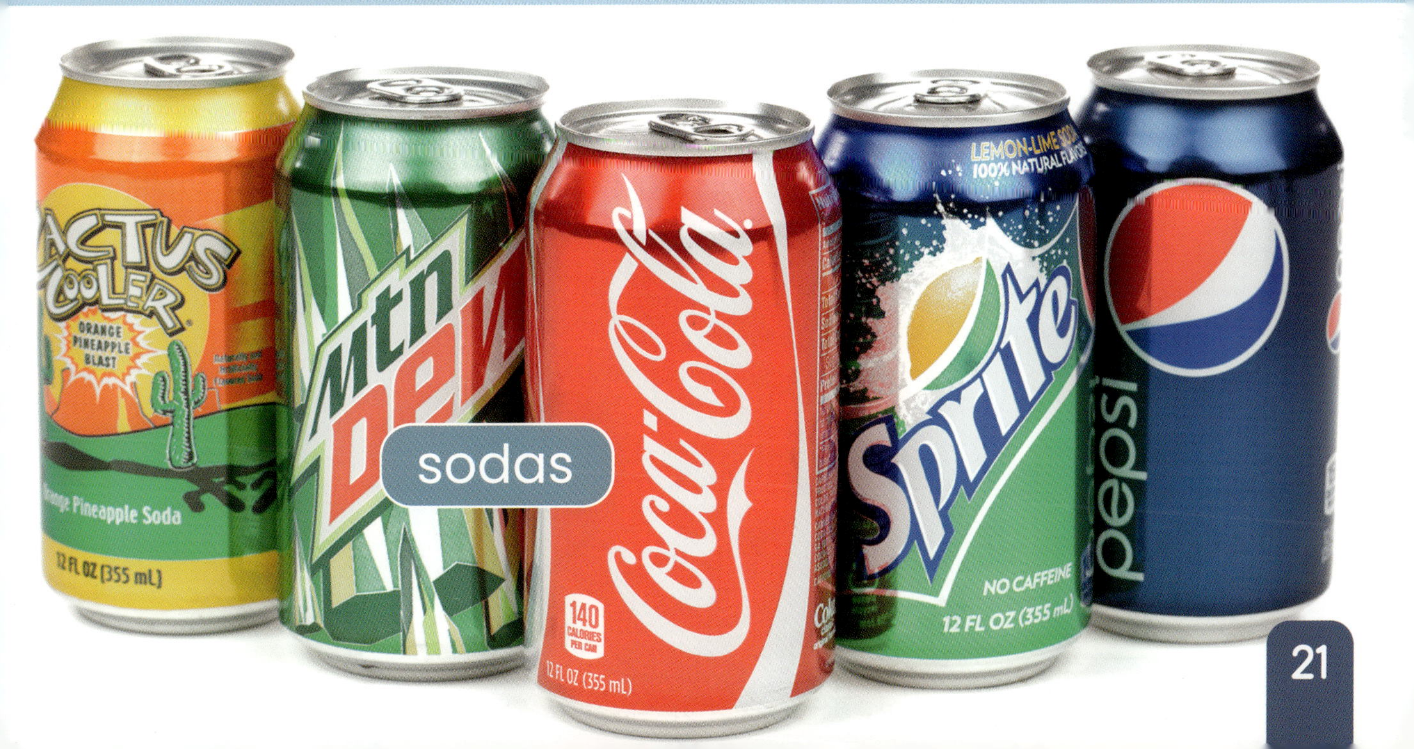
sodas
Orange Pineapple Soda
12 FL OZ (355 mL)
Coca-Cola
140 CALORIES PER CAN
12 FL OZ (355 mL)
Sprite
NO CAFFEINE
12 FL OZ (355 mL)
pepsi

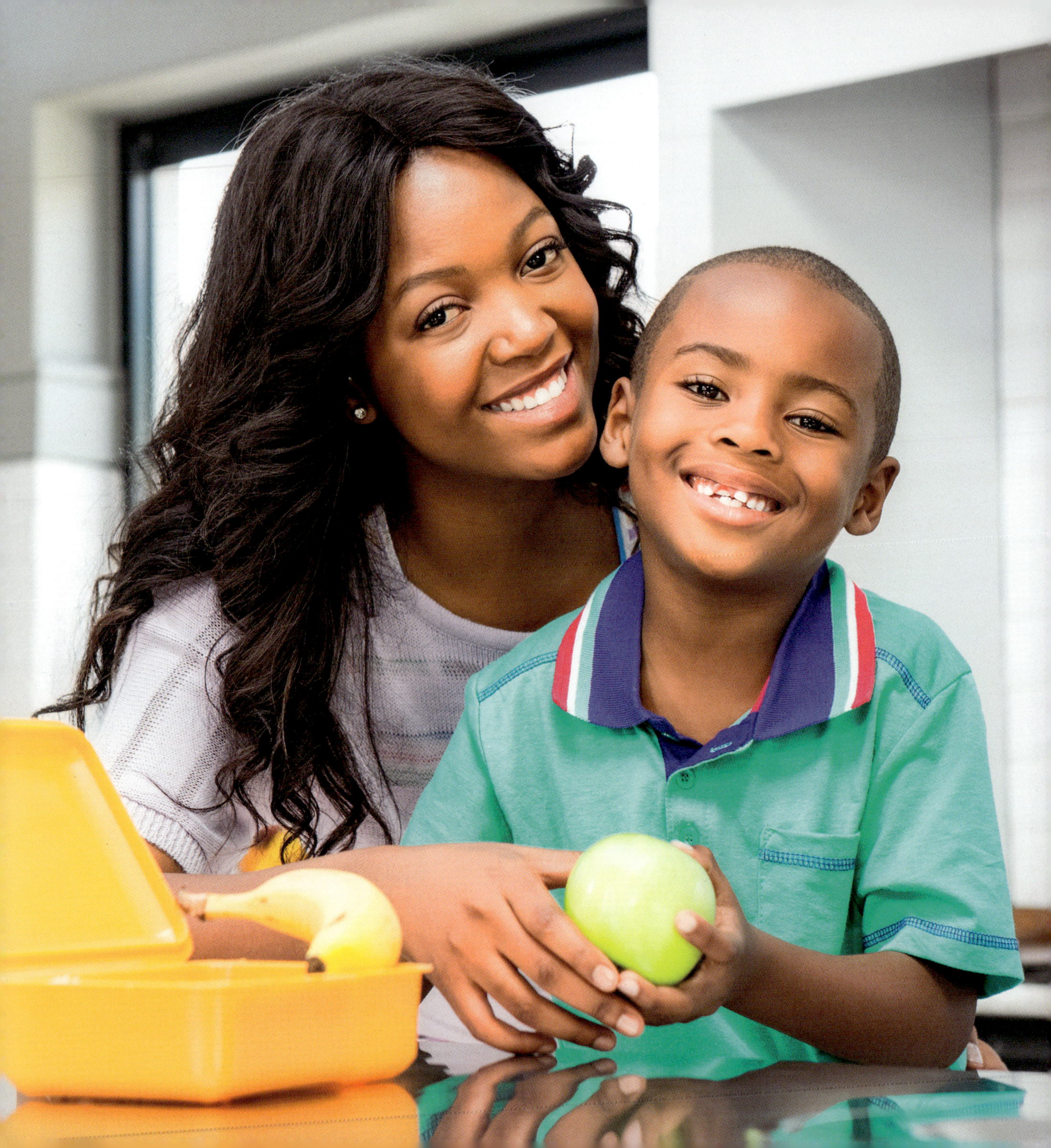

Eating Right

Lastly, listen to your body. Notice when you start feeling full, and then stop eating. Eating right will give you energy to enjoy your life.

Glossary

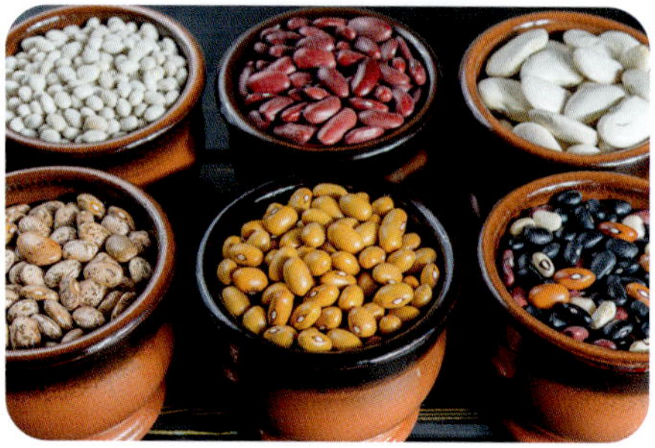

beans

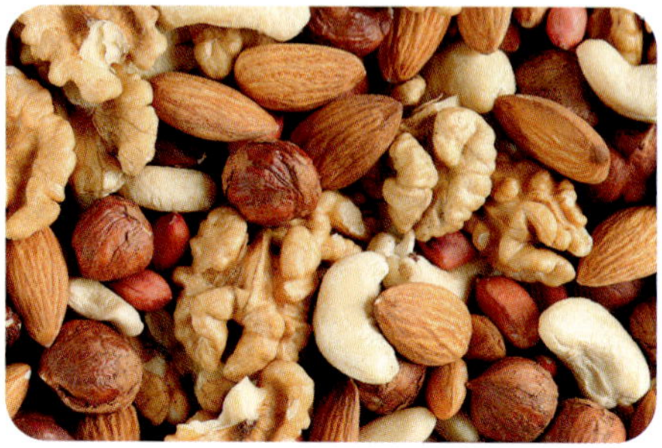

nuts

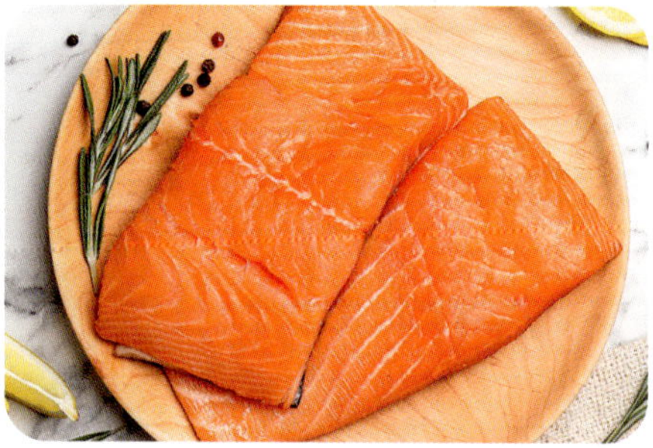

fish

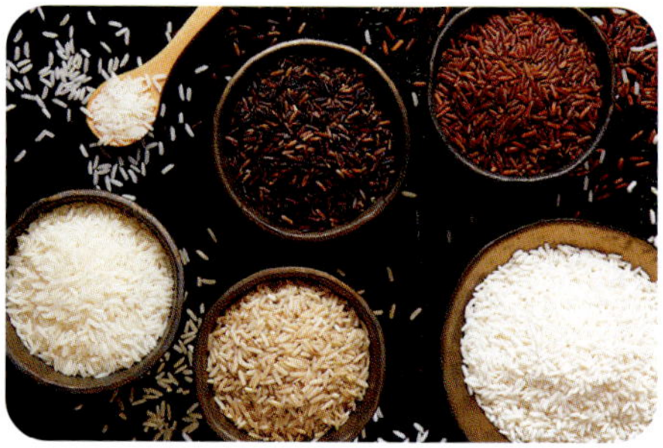

rice

Index